AF689737

COMMUNICATION STRATEGIES FOR EFFECTIVE LEADERSHIP AND TEAM MANAGEMENT

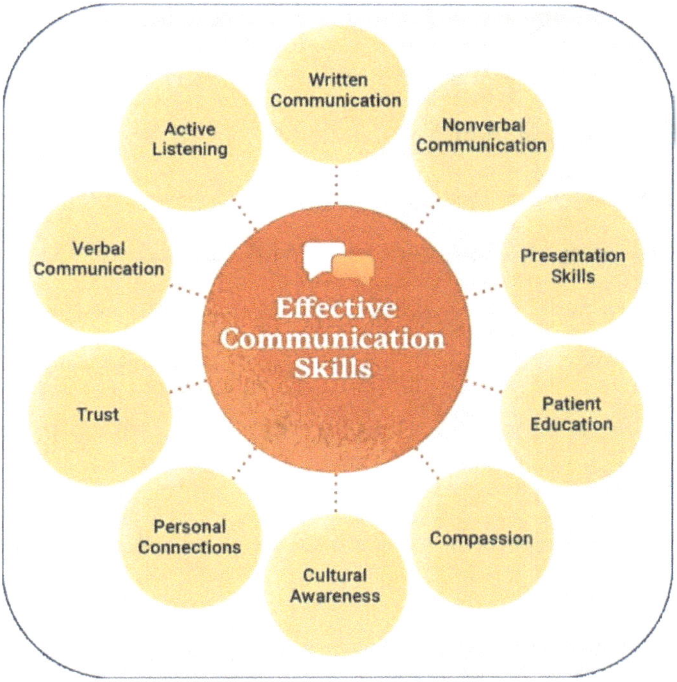

Table of Contents

COURSE OVERVIEW

This course is designed for healthcare professionals, particularly those in respiratory care, to enhance their communication skills, leadership abilities, and team management strategies. The course will cover essential aspects of leadership communication, conflict resolution, emotional intelligence, and effective team coordination, ensuring that respiratory care teams operate efficiently, collaboratively, and with a patient-centered focus.

COURSE OBJECTIVE

By the end of this course, healthcare providers specializing in respiratory care will be able to Understand the Role of Communication in Leadership and Team Management, Develop Key Communication Skills for Effective Leadership, Enhance Team Building and Collaboration through Communication, Master Crisis Communication and Leadership in Respiratory Care, Apply Patient-Centered Communication Strategies in Leadership, Utilize Technology to Improve Leadership Communication, Develop a Personalized Communication Strategy for Leadership Success, Address Ethical and Legal Considerations in Leadership Communication

By achieving these objectives, participants will gain the skills and confidence to lead effectively, foster teamwork, and enhance patient care through strategic communication in respiratory care settings.

INTRODUCTION

Effective leadership in respiratory care goes beyond clinical expertise it requires clear, ethical, and compassionate communication. Whether guiding a team, interacting with patients, or making high-stakes decisions, the ability to communicate effectively is essential for ensuring patient safety, staff cohesion, and positive healthcare outcomes.

This book is designed to provide respiratory care leaders, clinicians, and healthcare professionals with the tools needed to navigate the complexities of leadership communication and management

With case studies, and actionable strategies, this book serves as a comprehensive guide to mastering leadership communication and management in respiratory care. Whether you are a seasoned leader or an aspiring healthcare professional, these insights will help you build a strong, ethical, and effective communication framework ensuring better patient outcomes, a supportive workplace, and long-term success in your field.

Let's embark on this journey toward exceptional leadership and transformative communication and management in respiratory care.

MODULE ONE

THE ROLE OF COMMUNICATION IN LEADERSHIP AND TEAM MANAGEMENT IN RESPIRATORY CARE

Effective communication is the cornerstone of successful leadership and team management in respiratory care. In a fast-paced, high-stakes environment where healthcare providers must work cohesively to deliver optimal patient care, communication plays a critical role in decision-making, collaboration, and overall team efficiency. Leaders in respiratory care must cultivate a culture of open communication to ensure that patient outcomes are optimized, misunderstandings are minimized, and healthcare teams function seamlessly.

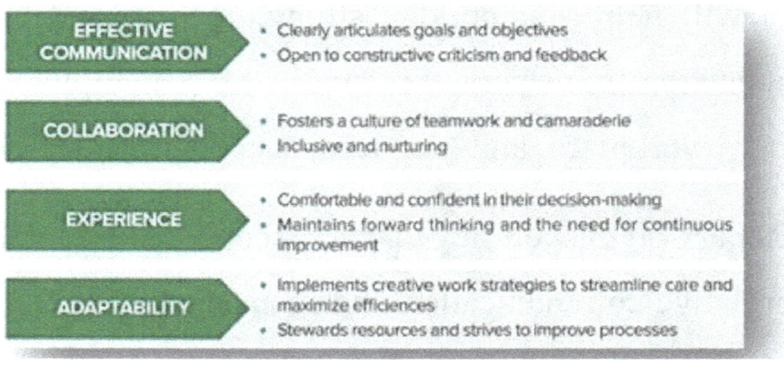

In this module, we will explore the significance of communication in leadership, its impact on patient care and team efficiency, common communication challenges in respiratory care, and strategies for fostering transparency in leadership.

UNDERSTANDING THE IMPORTANCE OF COMMUNICATION IN LEADERSHIP

Leadership is not just about decision-making or assigning tasks, it's about inspiring, guiding, and uniting a team toward a common goal. In respiratory care, this means ensuring clear, accurate, and timely communication to prevent errors and improve patient safety.

A leader's communication skills directly influence:

- How effectively a team collaborates
- The trust and morale within the department
- The ability to respond to emergencies and crises
- The clarity of protocols and standard procedures
- The ability to resolve conflicts and maintain a positive work environment

Key Communication Aspects in Leadership

- Clarity and Precision: Respiratory care involves critical tasks such as administering mechanical ventilation, managing airway support, and responding to respiratory emergencies. Miscommunication can result in serious medical errors. Leaders must convey clear, direct instructions to ensure patient safety.

- Active Listening: Effective leaders listen actively to their team's concerns, feedback, and suggestions. In respiratory care, this is essential when coordinating with physicians, nurses, and respiratory therapists to make informed treatment decisions.
- Adaptability in Communication: Different team members have varying communication styles. Leaders must adjust their approach based on the situation whether providing direct, urgent instructions in a crisis or fostering collaborative discussions during team meetings.
- Encouraging Open Dialogue: Creating an open-door policy where team members feel comfortable raising concerns without fear of judgment is crucial. In healthcare, withholding information due to fear or intimidation can lead to poor patient outcomes.
- Empathy and Emotional Intelligence: Leaders who communicate with empathy build stronger relationships within their teams. Recognizing when a team member is stressed or overwhelmed allows leaders to provide the

necessary support and maintain a healthy work environment.

THE IMPACT OF COMMUNICATION ON PATIENT OUTCOMES AND TEAM EFFICIENCY

Communication in respiratory care extends beyond team interactions, it directly affects patient outcomes. When healthcare teams communicate effectively, they reduce errors, enhance coordination, and ensure timely interventions for patients with respiratory conditions.

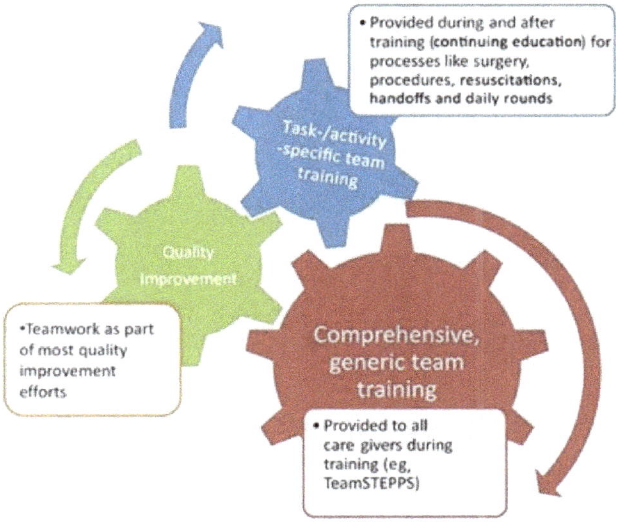

How Communication Affects Patient Outcomes

- Prevention of Medical Errors: Poor communication is one of the leading causes of adverse events in healthcare.

Misinterpretation of orders, incomplete patient handoffs, and unclear documentation can result in serious harm.

- Enhanced Patient Safety: When teams communicate clearly, medication administration, ventilation settings, and airway management procedures are executed with precision.
- Improved Patient Satisfaction: Patients and their families expect clear and compassionate communication regarding treatment plans. A well-informed patient is more likely to adhere to medical advice and experience positive health outcomes.
- Faster Emergency Response: In acute situations such as respiratory failure or asthma exacerbations, effective communication ensures quick decision-making and a coordinated response.

How Communication Enhances Team Efficiency

- Seamless Interdisciplinary Collaboration: Respiratory care involves working with physicians, nurses, anesthesiologists, and other specialists. Clear communication prevents duplication of efforts and ensures everyone is on the same page.
- Efficient Delegation of Tasks: Leaders must assign responsibilities clearly to avoid confusion. This is

especially important in high-pressure settings like ICUs and emergency departments.

- Reduction of Workplace Stress: Miscommunication can create tension and frustration among team members. Transparent communication helps reduce misunderstandings and foster a positive work culture.

COMMON COMMUNICATION CHALLENGES IN RESPIRATORY CARE SETTINGS

Despite its importance, communication in respiratory care is often challenged by various factors. Leaders must recognize and address these barriers to ensure a smooth workflow.

Key Challenges and How to Overcome Them

1. Time Constraints in High-Stress Environments
   - Respiratory therapists often work in fast-paced emergency settings where time is limited. Rushed communication can lead to misunderstandings and mistakes.
   - Solution: Use brief, standardized communication protocols such as SBAR (Situation, Background, Assessment, and Recommendation) to convey critical information efficiently.
2. Hierarchical Barriers

- Some team members may feel intimidated to speak up, especially in hierarchies where physicians or senior staff dominate discussions.
- Solution: Leaders should promote a collaborative, team-based approach where every voice is valued. Encourage team members to ask questions and provide input.

3. Multidisciplinary Communication Gaps
   - Respiratory care teams often interact with various departments. Miscommunication between specialties (e.g., ICU teams, anesthesia teams, and pulmonologists) can cause delays in care.
   - Solution: Implement structured handoff protocols and encourage interdisciplinary case discussions.
4. Emotional and Psychological Barriers
   - Healthcare professionals frequently deal with stress, fatigue, and emotional exhaustion, which can impair communication skills.
   - Solution: Leaders should recognize burnout symptoms and foster a supportive work environment through regular check-ins, debriefing sessions, and mental health resources.
5. Technological Challenges
   - The increasing reliance on electronic health records (EHRs) and telehealth has introduced new

communication barriers, such as documentation errors, misinterpretation of digital messages, and technical difficulties.

- Solution: Train staff on effective use of digital communication tools, ensuring clarity in written documentation and verifying information before acting.

THE LEADER'S ROLE IN FOSTERING AN OPEN AND TRANSPARENT COMMUNICATION CULTURE

Leaders must proactively create an environment where communication is valued, encouraged, and continuously improved.

Key Leadership Strategies

- Lead by Example: Model clear, respectful, and open communication in every interaction.
- Encourage Psychological Safety: Create an atmosphere where team members feel safe to express concerns, ask questions, and admit mistakes without fear of punishment.
- Use Regular Team Meetings: Conduct structured huddles and debriefings to discuss patient cases, address challenges, and improve workflow.

- Provide Constructive Feedback: Feedback should be timely, specific, and solution-focused, helping team members grow without discouragement.
- Utilize Communication Training: Offer ongoing training sessions on active listening, conflict resolution, and effective handoff techniques.

THE RELATIONSHIP BETWEEN COMMUNICATION AND DECISION-MAKING

Effective communication is central to strong leadership decision-making in respiratory care.

How Communication Enhances Decision-Making

- Ensures Informed Choices: Leaders need accurate, timely information from their teams to make the best clinical and operational decisions.
- Promotes Collaboration: Decision-making should involve input from multiple perspectives, fostering well-rounded solutions.
- Minimizes Risk and Uncertainty: Open discussions help leaders identify potential issues early and create proactive strategies.

Decision-Making Models in Healthcare

- Shared Decision-Making (SDM): Engages both healthcare providers and patients in treatment decisions.
- Evidence-Based Decision-Making: Utilizes research and clinical data to guide respiratory care plans.

DISCUSSION QUESTIONS

- How does effective communication impact patient care in respiratory therapy?
- What are some common communication barriers that respiratory care leaders face, and how can they be overcome?

MODULE TWO

KEY COMMUNICATION SKILLS FOR EFFECTIVE LEADERSHIP IN RESPIRATORY CARE

Effective communication skills are essential for leaders in respiratory care, ensuring smooth team collaboration, patient safety, and high-quality care. Leadership is not just about making decisions but also about how well a leader conveys those decisions, fosters understanding, and builds a strong, cooperative team.

- Pay attention
  - Make eye contact
  - Observe body language (theirs)
  - Remove distractions
- Show that you are listening
  - Your body language
  - Encouraging comments
- Provide feedback
  - Reflective statements
  - Clarify points
- Defer judgment
  - Listen to the "whole story"
  - Don't interrupt
- Respond appropriately
  - Be candid in your response

Respiratory care professionals work in fast-paced, high-pressure environments where communication must be clear, empathetic, and effective to ensure optimal patient outcomes and team efficiency. This module explores the five key communication skills that every respiratory care leader should master: active listening, verbal vs. non-verbal communication, empathy, feedback techniques, and assertiveness.

ACTIVE LISTENING: ENHANCING UNDERSTANDING AND RAPPORT

What Is Active Listening?

Active listening is the ability to fully concentrate, understand, respond, and remember what is being said. Unlike passive listening, which involves merely hearing words, active listening requires engagement and comprehension.

In respiratory care, active listening is crucial for leaders because they must:

- Understand the concerns of their team members
- Ensure that instructions are clear and followed correctly
- Enhance patient-provider interactions
- Recognize underlying issues in communication breakdowns

Key Elements of Active Listening

- Maintaining Eye Contact: This shows engagement and attentiveness in both team and patient interactions.
- Paraphrasing and Summarizing: Repeating or summarizing what was said helps confirm understanding (e.g., "So you're saying that the ventilator settings need adjustment for better oxygenation?").
- Asking Open-Ended Questions: Encourages deeper discussions and clarifications (e.g., "Can you tell me more about your concerns regarding the new protocol?").
- Avoiding Interruptions: Shows respect and genuine interest in the conversation.
- Providing Verbal and Non-Verbal Feedback: Nods, affirmations, and facial expressions help indicate engagement and understanding.

The Role of Active Listening in Leadership

A respiratory care leader who actively listens:

- Builds trust within the team
- Reduces miscommunication and errors
- Encourages open discussions, leading to problem-solving
- Ensures team members feel heard and valued

Example Scenario:

A respiratory therapist raises concerns about a new mechanical ventilation protocol. Instead of dismissing them, the leader listens attentively, asks clarifying questions, and summarizes their concerns. As a result, the team collaborates to refine the protocol, improving both workflow and patient care.

VERBAL VS. NON-VERBAL COMMUNICATION IN HEALTHCARE SETTINGS

Verbal Communication

Verbal communication in respiratory care leadership involves spoken words, tone, and clarity of speech. This includes:

- Giving clear instructions to team members
- Explaining procedures to patients
- Collaborating with interdisciplinary teams

Best Practices for Verbal Communication:

- Use Simple, Concise Language: Avoid jargon when speaking to patients or junior staff.
- Adjust Tone and Volume: Speak calmly in high-stress situations to maintain clarity.

- Use Structured Communication Protocols: Methods like SBAR (Situation, Background, Assessment, and Recommendation) help ensure clarity.

Non-Verbal Communication

Non-verbal communication includes body language, facial expressions, gestures, and eye contact. In leadership, non-verbal cues can reinforce or contradict spoken words.

Key Non-Verbal Communication Tips:

- Maintain Open Body Language: Crossed arms can signal defensiveness, while an open posture shows receptiveness.
- Use Appropriate Facial Expressions: A reassuring smile can ease a patient's anxiety.
- Observe Team Members' Non-Verbal Cues: Recognizing when a team member looks overwhelmed allows leaders to intervene with support.

Example Scenario:

A respiratory care leader explains a new intubation procedure in an ICU meeting. If they speak confidently but avoid eye contact and have a closed posture, their team may perceive uncertainty or lack of engagement, impacting team confidence.

COMMUNICATING WITH EMPATHY AND CLARITY IN STRESSFUL SITUATIONS

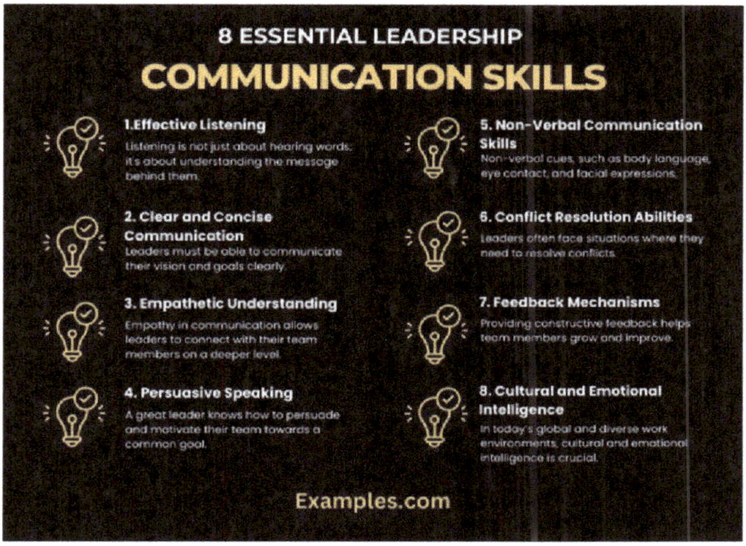

Why Is Empathy Important in Respiratory Care?

Empathy allows leaders to connect with their team members and patients on an emotional level. In high-stress environments like ICUs, emotional intelligence is essential to maintain a supportive atmosphere.

Key Components of Empathetic Communication:

- Acknowledgment: Recognizing and validating the feelings of others (e.g., "I understand this new policy is challenging. Let's discuss how we can make it work.").
- Active Engagement: Showing interest in the concerns of patients and team members.

- Calm and Reassuring Speech: Speaking in a composed manner helps de-escalate stress.

Example Scenario:

A family member is distressed about their loved one's ventilator settings. A respiratory leader who listens, explains clearly, and reassures them with empathy fosters trust and collaboration in care decisions.

FEEDBACK TECHNIQUES FOR IMPROVING TEAM PERFORMANCE

The Importance of Constructive Feedback

Effective leaders provide regular feedback to help their teams grow. Feedback should be timely, specific, and constructive rather than critical.

Best Practices for Effective Feedback:

- Use the "Sandwich Method": Start with positive feedback, provide constructive suggestions, and end with encouragement.
- Be Specific: Instead of saying, "You need to be more careful," say, "Double-check ventilator settings before intubation to avoid errors."
- Encourage Two-Way Dialogue: Allow team members to discuss their challenges and solutions.

Example Scenario:

A leader notices a respiratory therapist struggling with a new protocol. Instead of criticizing, they offer guidance, demonstrate proper techniques, and encourage open discussion, leading to improved confidence and performance.

THE ROLE OF ASSERTIVENESS IN LEADERSHIP COMMUNICATION

What Is Assertive Communication?

Assertiveness is the ability to express one's thoughts, needs, and expectations clearly and confidently, without aggression or passivity.

Why Is Assertiveness Important in Respiratory Care?

- Ensures patient safety by speaking up about concerns
- Improves interdisciplinary collaboration
- Helps leaders maintain authority while fostering respect

Techniques for Assertive Communication:

- Use "I" Statements: Instead of blaming, say, "I need everyone to double-check oxygen levels before extubation."
- Be Direct but Respectful: Clearly state expectations while maintaining a professional and respectful tone.

- Set Boundaries: Leaders should clearly define roles and responsibilities to prevent burnout.

Example Scenario:

A physician requests an unnecessary respiratory treatment. A confident leader says, "I understand your concern, but based on the latest protocol, this patient does not require that intervention." This ensures evidence-based decision-making while maintaining professionalism.

Effective leadership in respiratory care depends on strong communication skills. Active listening, verbal and non-verbal communication, empathetic interactions, constructive feedback, and assertiveness all contribute to a well-functioning team and improved patient outcomes.

Discussion Questions:

- How can respiratory care leaders balance assertiveness with empathy when making critical decisions?
- What strategies can be used to ensure team members feel comfortable providing feedback to leadership?

MODULE THREE

BUILDING STRONG TEAMS THROUGH COMMUNICATION

A successful respiratory care team is built on trust, collaboration, and effective communication. The ability of a leader to foster teamwork directly impacts patient care, staff morale, and overall efficiency in respiratory therapy units. Poor communication can lead to misunderstandings, inefficiencies, and even medical errors.

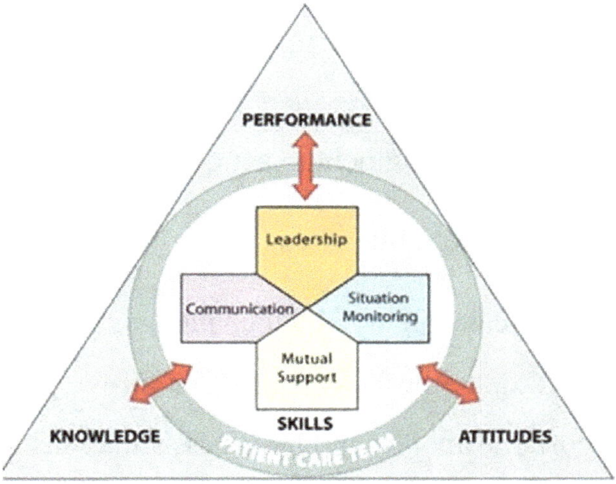

This module explores five critical aspects of team-building through communication:

- Trust and collaboration
- Strategies to enhance team cohesion

- Conflict prevention and resolution
- Task delegation
- Interdisciplinary communication

A respiratory care leader who masters these elements creates a supportive environment where team members feel valued, respected, and empowered to provide the best possible care.

THE IMPORTANCE OF TRUST AND COLLABORATION IN TEAM BUILDING

Why Is Trust Essential in Respiratory Care Teams?

Trust is the foundation of teamwork in healthcare. In a high-pressure setting, such as an ICU or emergency department, respiratory therapists, nurses, and physicians must trust each other's expertise and judgment to act quickly and efficiently.

A trusting team is more likely to:

- Communicate openly about challenges and concerns.
- Rely on each other's strengths to improve patient care.
- Support one another in high-stress situations.

How Leaders Can Build Trust Through Communication

- Transparency: Share relevant information openly, ensuring that all team members are on the same page. For example, if a new ventilation protocol is being implemented, leaders should clearly explain why the change is occurring and how it benefits both patients and staff.

- Accountability: Acknowledge mistakes and take responsibility. If a leader makes an error in decision-making, admitting it fosters honesty and encourages others to take responsibility as well.
- Consistency: Being reliable and following through on commitments reinforces a leader's credibility. For example, if a leader promises additional training on new oxygenation procedures, they should ensure it happens.

Collaboration: The Key to Team Success

Collaboration in respiratory care involves team members working together effectively to enhance patient care. Leaders must encourage a shared decision-making approach, where every voice is heard and valued.

Example: In a case of acute respiratory distress syndrome (ARDS), a multidisciplinary approach involving respiratory therapists, pulmonologists, ICU nurses, and radiologists ensures that all aspects of the patient's care are addressed. A collaborative environment enables better decision-making and improves patient survival rates.

STRATEGIES TO ENHANCE TEAM COHESION THROUGH COMMUNICATION

Team cohesion refers to how well team members work together toward a common goal. A well-cohesive respiratory care team is more efficient, motivated, and resilient under pressure.

Communication Strategies to Strengthen Team Cohesion

1. Regular Team Meetings

- Conduct daily or weekly huddles to discuss patient care updates, challenges, and expectations.
- Allow open discussions where team members voice concerns and share insights.

2. Establish a Culture of Psychological Safety

- Team members should feel safe to express opinions without fear of criticism or judgment.
- Leaders should validate concerns and encourage constructive discussions.

3. Encourage Peer-to-Peer Communication

- Promote an environment where team members consult and support each other.
- Example: A senior respiratory therapist mentoring a new staff member strengthens both skill development and team unity.

4. Use Technology to Improve Communication
    - Implement tools like secure messaging apps for quick updates on patient care.
    - Use digital dashboards to keep track of ventilator settings, patient progress, and workload distribution.
5. Foster Inclusivity and Team Identity
    - Recognize and celebrate team achievements.
    - Organize team-building activities, such as case study discussions, workshops, or informal gatherings.

THE ROLE OF A LEADER IN CONFLICT PREVENTION AND RESOLUTION

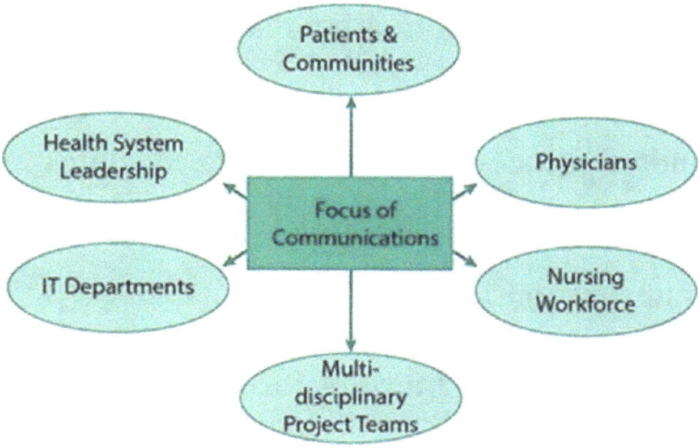

Understanding Conflict in Respiratory Care Teams

Conflicts can arise due to:

- Miscommunication between team members (e.g., misunderstanding verbal orders).

- Differences in decision-making approaches (e.g., a therapist and physician disagreeing on an intubation strategy).
- Workload imbalance, leading to resentment and frustration.

Conflict Prevention Strategies

- Set Clear Expectations: Clearly define roles, responsibilities, and protocols to prevent misunderstandings.
- Encourage Open Dialogue: If a therapist disagrees with a physician's approach, a leader should facilitate a respectful discussion rather than let tensions escalate.
- Develop Conflict Resolution Protocols: Establish a standard process for addressing disputes, such as a mediation step before escalating conflicts to administration.

Conflict Resolution Techniques for Leaders

- Active Mediation: Listen to both sides without bias and guide the team toward a mutual resolution.
- Reframing the Issue: Shift the focus from personal grievances to the shared goal of patient care.

- Encourage a Solutions-Oriented Approach: Instead of assigning blame, focus on what can be improved moving forward.

Example: A respiratory therapist and nurse disagree on a patient's suctioning schedule. A strong leader facilitates a discussion on evidence-based practices, ensuring both parties feel heard while reinforcing patient-centered care as the priority.

USING EFFECTIVE COMMUNICATION TO DELEGATE TASKS EFFICIENTLY

Delegation is a core leadership skill that ensures workload distribution is fair and effective. Poor delegation leads to burnout, errors, and reduced morale.

Best Practices for Delegating Tasks in Respiratory Care

1. Assess Team Strengths and Skills
   - Assign tasks based on individual expertise. For example, a therapist with advanced ventilator management skills can oversee complex ventilator setups.
   - Rotate tasks to ensure skill development and prevent monotony.
2. Provide Clear Instructions

- Be specific when assigning tasks: "I need you to conduct ABG analysis and report back within 30 minutes" is clearer than "Check the patient's blood gases."

Ensure Accountability Without Micromanaging

- Trust team members to complete their tasks, but provide opportunities for questions or clarifications.
- Encourage self-reporting on task completion and challenges encountered.

Example: A leader overseeing a post-COVID-19 pulmonary rehab unit delegates spirometry testing to one therapist and patient education on breathing exercises to another, ensuring efficient use of expertise.

THE IMPACT OF INTERDISCIPLINARY COMMUNICATION IN RESPIRATORY CARE

Respiratory care leaders must coordinate with other healthcare professionals, including nurses, physicians, physical therapists, and dietitians. Interdisciplinary communication ensures holistic patient care.

Why Is Interdisciplinary Communication Critical?

- Reduces Medical Errors: Miscommunication between departments is a leading cause of preventable errors.

- Enhances Patient Outcomes: Coordinated efforts improve efficiency in treatment planning and execution.
- Fosters a Teamwork Culture: Encourages mutual respect and shared learning.

Strategies for Effective Interdisciplinary Communication

- Standardized Communication Protocols (e.g., SBAR - Situation, Background, Assessment, and Recommendation).
- Interdisciplinary Rounds to ensure all care providers are aligned.
- Encouraging Direct Collaboration (e.g., having a respiratory therapist discuss treatment options directly with pulmonologists).

Example: In a mechanically ventilated patient, effective communication between the respiratory therapist, intensivist, and nutritionist ensures appropriate sedation levels, ventilator weaning strategies, and nutritional support, leading to faster recovery.

Building strong teams in respiratory care requires a leader to foster trust, communication, and collaboration. Effective delegation, conflict resolution, and interdisciplinary coordination are essential for high-functioning teams and better patient outcomes.

DISCUSSION QUESTIONS:

- What are the biggest challenges respiratory care teams face in interdisciplinary communication, and how can leaders address them?
- How can respiratory care leaders create a work environment where team members feel comfortable addressing conflicts constructively?

MODULE FOUR

CRISIS COMMUNICATION AND LEADERSHIP IN RESPIRATORY CARE

Crisis situations in respiratory care demand clear, rapid, and effective communication. Whether responding to a mass casualty event, a sudden ICU surge, or a ventilator shortage, leaders must guide their teams with confidence, make quick decisions, and keep all stakeholders informed.

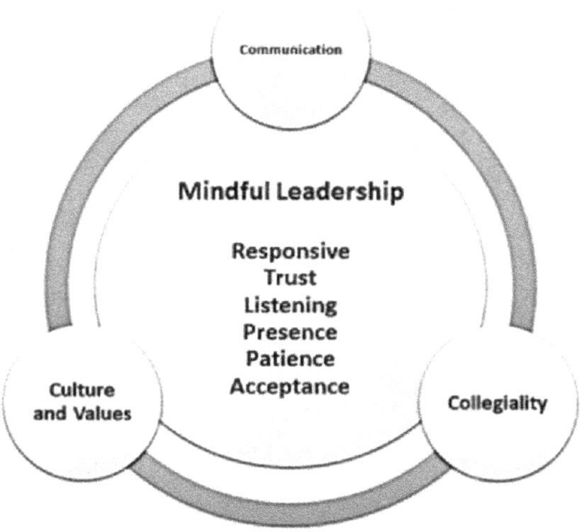

This module covers five critical aspects of crisis communication:

- Best practices for communicating during emergencies
- The leader's role in crisis management

- Decision-making under pressure
- Handling public relations and media inquiries
- Post-crisis debriefing

Mastering these elements ensures patient safety, team efficiency, and public trust in times of crisis.

COMMUNICATING DURING EMERGENCIES: BEST PRACTICES

Why Is Emergency Communication Critical?

Emergencies such as cardiac arrests, mass casualty incidents, or sudden outbreaks require precise and fast communication. Delays or miscommunication can lead to worsening patient conditions, treatment errors, and staff confusion.

Best Practices for Emergency Communication

1. Use Clear, Direct, and Concise Language

In high-stress situations, long explanations create confusion. Leaders must use short, action-oriented phrases:

- Instead of: "Can someone check on the ventilator settings when they have time?"
- Say: "John, check the ventilator settings now and report back in two minutes."

2. Implement the Chain of Command

A clear hierarchy ensures information flows correctly. In a crisis, every team member should know:

- Who to report to
- Who is making final decisions
- How to escalate issues

Example: In a ventilator failure situation, the respiratory therapy lead should immediately notify ICU physicians, while an assistant checks alternative oxygenation options.

3. Utilize Emergency Communication Systems

- Overhead paging systems for immediate hospital-wide alerts.
- Radios or secure mobile apps for real-time coordination between departments.
- Color-coded emergency alerts to ensure rapid response without verbal delays.

4. Assign Specific Roles in Crisis Situations

- One person manages intubations, another monitors oxygen levels, and a third contacts necessary departments.
- Having pre-defined roles prevents panic and streamlines emergency actions.

5. Ensure Staff is Trained in Crisis Communication

- Regular drills, simulations, and case reviews enhance team preparedness.

THE ROLE OF A LEADER IN CRISIS MANAGEMENT

Key Responsibilities of a Leader in a Crisis

- Maintaining composure: A leader's demeanor influences the team's response.
- Providing clear direction: Teams rely on concise instructions and quick decisions.
- Prioritizing patient safety: Leaders triage and allocate resources to protect lives.
- Coordinating with other departments: A respiratory care leader must communicate with ICU teams, hospital administration, and emergency personnel.
- Keeping morale high: A leader motivates the team and reduces panic.

How Leaders Can Stay Effective Under Pressure

- Use a calm, assertive tone: Panic spreads quickly staying composed helps keep the team focused.
- Ensure rapid but thoughtful decision-making: Leaders must weigh risks, prioritize tasks, and adapt quickly.
- Encourage teamwork: Delegate tasks efficiently so that no individual becomes overwhelmed.

Example: During a hospital-wide oxygen shortage, a respiratory therapy leader must:

- Assess oxygen reserves and prioritize patients based on severity.
- Communicate with administration for emergency oxygen delivery.
- Coordinate with ICU and ER teams to minimize unnecessary oxygen usage.

DECISION-MAKING UNDER PRESSURE: COMMUNICATION STRATEGIES

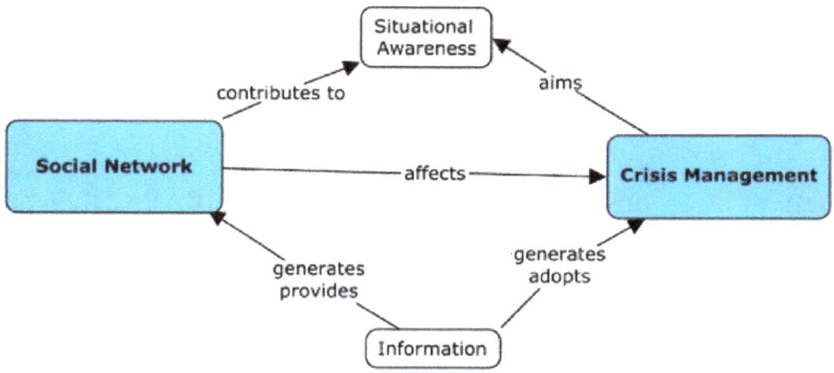

The Challenge of High-Stakes Decision-Making

Decisions made under crisis conditions carry significant risks. Poor communication can lead to fatal errors.

Effective Decision-Making Strategies

1. Prioritize Based on Medical Urgency

In a crisis, leaders must triage effectively:

- High priority: Patients needing immediate intubation.
- Medium priority: Patients who can be stabilized with non-invasive oxygen.
- Lower priority: Patients who are improving and need minimal intervention.

2. Use the SBAR Framework for Quick Decision Communication

- Situation: Clearly state the issue.
- Background: Provide relevant patient history.
- Assessment: Explain the current condition.
- Recommendation: Suggest the best course of action.

Example:

"Patient X is desaturating at 85% despite BiPAP. They have severe COPD. We need to prepare for intubation now."

3. Avoid Decision Fatigue

- Rotate leadership roles during prolonged crises to prevent burnout.
- Ensure breaks so that leaders remain sharp.

HANDLING PUBLIC RELATIONS AND MEDIA INQUIRIES IN HEALTHCARE CRISES

Why Is Public Communication Important?

In major crises (e.g., pandemics, hospital-wide equipment failures), patients, families, and the public demand accurate information. Poor handling of public relations can lead to panic, misinformation, and loss of trust in the healthcare system.

Best Practices for Crisis Public Communication

1. Designate a Spokesperson
    - The hospital or healthcare institution should have a trained representative (often a senior leader).
    - Avoid multiple sources giving conflicting statements.
2. Use Simple and Reassuring Language
    - Avoid medical jargon: Instead of "Oxygen saturation levels are suboptimal," say, "We are taking every step to ensure patients receive the oxygen they need."
    - Acknowledge concerns but emphasize solutions.
3. Maintain Transparency
    - Be honest about what is known and what is being done.
    - Example: "We are experiencing a ventilator shortage, but additional units are being delivered within the hour."
4. Control the Spread of Misinformation

- Provide regular updates through hospital websites, press releases, or social media.
- Correct false rumors promptly and professionally.

CRISIS DEBRIEFING: IMPROVING FUTURE RESPONSES

Why Is Post-Crisis Evaluation Necessary?

After a crisis, reflecting on what went well and what needs improvement helps teams prepare for future emergencies.

Steps for an Effective Debriefing Process

1. Conduct a Team Meeting
    - Gather all staff involved and discuss strengths and weaknesses in the response.
    - Encourage open discussion without assigning blame.
2. Identify Key Challenges
    - Were there delays in communication?
    - Were roles and responsibilities clear?
    - Did staff have enough training to handle the crisis?
3. Develop an Improvement Plan
    - Implement new protocols based on identified weaknesses.
    - Schedule additional training sessions if needed.
4. Provide Emotional Support for Staff

- Crises can lead to burnout, anxiety, and PTSD in healthcare workers.
- Offer counseling, peer support groups, or structured mental health resources.

Example: After a mass casualty event, debriefing revealed that a lack of a clear patient tracking system caused confusion. As a result, the hospital introduced digital triage boards for future incidents.

Crisis communication in respiratory care requires preparation, composure, and strategic leadership. Leaders must guide their teams efficiently, communicate with the public responsibly, and continuously improve emergency response strategies.

Discussion Questions:

- How can respiratory therapy leaders prepare their teams for an unpredictable crisis?
- What strategies can hospitals use to improve public trust during a crisis?
- How can leaders balance rapid decision-making with patient safety under pressure?

MODULE FIVE

PATIENT-CENTERED COMMUNICATION AND LEADERSHIP IN RESPIRATORY CARE

Effective communication is a cornerstone of patient-centered care. In respiratory therapy, clear and compassionate communication not only enhances patient trust and compliance but also improves clinical outcomes. A leader in respiratory care must bridge the gap between medical expertise and patient understanding, ensuring that every patient receives safe, respectful, and personalized care.

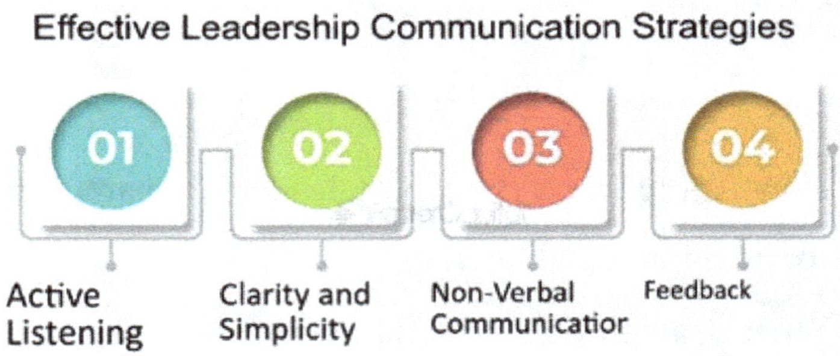

This module explores five key aspects of patient-centered communication in respiratory care:

- The leader's role in patient communication
- Ensuring patient safety through clear communication

- Cultural competency and diversity in patient interactions
- Handling difficult conversations with patients and families
- Using shared decision-making to improve patient outcomes

Mastering these elements ensures higher patient satisfaction, better adherence to treatment, and improved overall care quality.

THE LEADER'S ROLE IN PATIENT COMMUNICATION

Why is Patient Communication a Leadership Responsibility?

Leaders in respiratory care whether respiratory therapists, physicians, or department heads set the tone for communication practices. Their approach directly influences how their teams interact with patients.

Key Responsibilities of a Leader in Patient Communication

1. Setting Communication Standards

Leaders must ensure that every team member:

- Uses clear, jargon-free language.
- Engages in active listening to understand patient concerns.

- Provides accurate and consistent information.

2. Training and Mentorship

Leaders should train junior staff on patient communication techniques, including:

- Breaking down complex medical information into easy-to-understand explanations.
- Using nonverbal cues (eye contact, tone, body language) to convey empathy.
- Encouraging questions to ensure patient understanding.

3. Modeling Compassionate Care

Patients with chronic respiratory diseases (e.g., COPD, asthma) often experience fear and anxiety about their condition. Leaders must demonstrate empathy and patience when discussing:

- Prognosis and treatment plans.
- Long-term disease management.
- Lifestyle adjustments for respiratory health.

4. Advocating for Patient Needs

Leaders ensure that patients' voices are heard and respected in treatment decisions. This involves:

- Addressing barriers to care (e.g., language, health literacy).

- Coordinating with multidisciplinary teams to align treatment goals.
- Encouraging family involvement in care discussions.

ENSURING PATIENT SAFETY THROUGH CLEAR COMMUNICATION

How Can Poor Communication Compromise Patient Safety?

Miscommunication in healthcare leads to medication errors, delayed treatments, and procedural mistakes. In respiratory care, unclear communication can result in oxygen mismanagement, ventilator misuse, or improper inhaler technique.

Strategies to Improve Patient Safety Through Communication

1. Use Teach-Back Methods

After explaining a treatment or procedure, ask the patient to repeat the instructions in their own words.

Example: Instead of simply asking, "Do you understand how to use the inhaler?" say,

"Can you show me how you'll use your inhaler at home?"

2. Confirm Understanding with Written and Visual Aids

Provide illustrated guides for complex respiratory therapies.

Use multilingual materials to ensure non-English-speaking patients understand.

Offer step-by-step video tutorials for using CPAP machines or nebulizers.

3. Standardize Communication in Handovers

When transferring patient care, ensure critical respiratory details are clearly conveyed to the next provider:

Oxygen requirements

- Ventilator settings
- Current respiratory treatments

Allergy history

Using structured formats like SBAR (Situation, Background, Assessment, and Recommendation) prevents miscommunication.

CULTURAL COMPETENCY AND DIVERSITY IN PATIENT INTERACTIONS

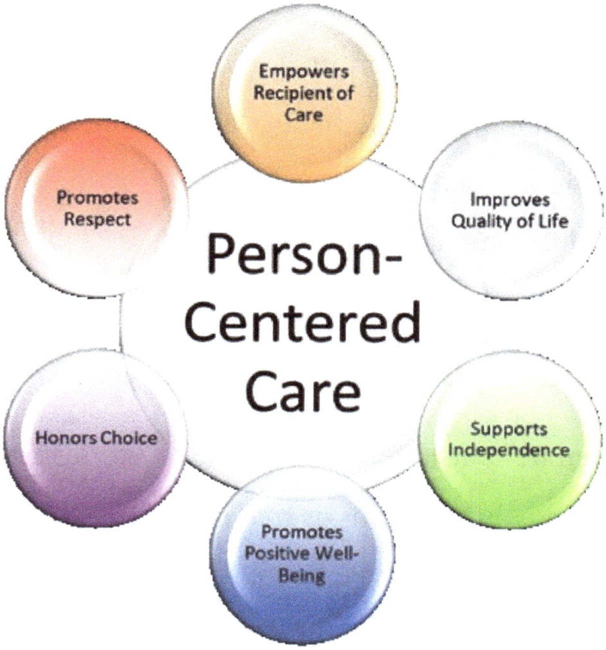

Empowers Recipient of Care
Improves Quality of Life
Supports Independence
Promotes Positive Well-Being
Honors Choice
Promotes Respect
Person-Centered Care

Why is Cultural Competency Important in Respiratory Care?

Patients come from diverse backgrounds, with different beliefs, languages, and health perceptions. Culturally competent communication ensures equitable care for all patients.

Best Practices for Culturally Sensitive Communication

1. Learn About Cultural Beliefs on Respiratory Health

Some cultures may:

- Prefer herbal remedies over inhalers.
- Have mistrust of Western medicine due to past experiences.
- Avoid discussing terminal illnesses openly.
- Understanding these beliefs helps tailor communication and build trust.

2. Use Professional Interpreters

Avoid using family members as translators—they may alter medical details. A trained medical interpreter ensures:

- Accurate translations of symptoms and instructions.
- Patient confidentiality is maintained.

3. Respect Religious and Personal Preferences

- Some Muslim patients may fast during Ramadan, affecting medication timing.
- Certain Indigenous groups prioritize holistic healing over pharmaceuticals.
- Jehovah's Witness patients may refuse blood transfusions.

Respecting these preferences while providing safe alternatives fosters trust and adherence.

4. Avoid Making Assumptions

- Do not assume health literacy based on education level.

- Ask open-ended questions to understand individual preferences.

HANDLING DIFFICULT CONVERSATIONS WITH PATIENTS AND FAMILIES

Common Difficult Conversations in Respiratory Care

- Telling a patient they need long-term oxygen therapy.
- Discussing terminal diagnoses, like end-stage COPD.
- Explaining why a treatment isn't working as expected.

Best Practices for Difficult Conversations

1. Use Empathy and Active Listening
   - Acknowledge emotions: "I can see this is overwhelming for you."
   - Pause and give time for the patient to process information.

2. Be Honest but Compassionate
   - Instead of: "Your lungs are too damaged, and there's nothing we can do."
   - Say: "Your condition has progressed, but we will focus on keeping you comfortable and improving your quality of life."

3. Involve Families in End-of-Life Discussions
   - Ask the patient about advanced care directives early.

- Provide palliative care options with dignity.

USING SHARED DECISION-MAKING TO IMPROVE PATIENT OUTCOMES

What is Shared Decision-Making?

Shared decision-making (SDM) is a collaborative process where:

- Clinicians provide evidence-based treatment options.
- Patients share their values and preferences.
- A joint decision is made that respects patient autonomy.

How SDM Benefits Respiratory Care

- Increases treatment adherence.
- Reduces patient anxiety by giving them control.
- Improves satisfaction and trust in medical care.

Steps to Implement Shared Decision-Making

1. Present All Options Clearly

For a COPD patient:

"You have two options: a CPAP machine at night or an alternative BiPAP therapy. Let's discuss the pros and cons of each."

2. Use Decision Aids

Visual charts comparing different treatments.

Risk-benefit scales to help patients weigh choices.

3. Empower Patients to Ask Questions

Encourage: “What concerns do you have about this treatment?”

Allow time for patients to discuss options with family.

MODULE SIX

DEVELOPING A COMMUNICATION STRATEGY FOR LEADERSHIP SUCCESS

One of the most critical skills for a successful leader is effective communication. Whether managing a respiratory care team, a healthcare department, or a corporate setting, a leader's ability to communicate clearly, inspire confidence, and foster collaboration determines team success.

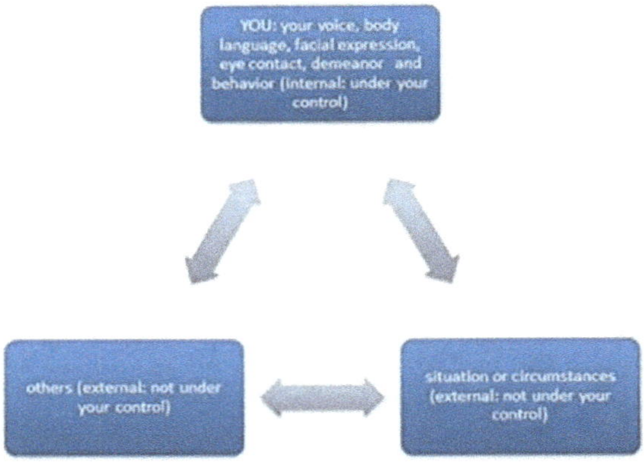

A well-structured communication strategy is essential to ensure team alignment with organizational goals, prevent misunderstandings that lead to inefficiency, enhance team morale and engagement, and develop a culture of continuous improvement.

This module explores how leaders can develop and implement a successful communication strategy through creating a personal leadership communication plan, setting communication goals for team success, coaching and mentoring for communication improvement, evaluating team communication effectiveness, continuous learning and adaptation in leadership communication.

CREATING A PERSONAL LEADERSHIP COMMUNICATION PLAN

Why Every Leader Needs a Communication Plan

A personal leadership communication plan helps leaders:

- Define their communication strengths and weaknesses.
- Establish a clear, authentic leadership voice.
- Ensure consistency in messaging across different situations.
- Align their communication style with their leadership values.

Steps to Develop a Personal Communication Plan

1. Self-Assessment: Identifying Strengths and Weaknesses

Begin by evaluating how you currently communicate with your team. Ask yourself:

- Do I communicate clearly and concisely?
- Am I approachable and open to feedback?
- Do I adjust my communication style based on the situation?
- Am I an active listener?

Using tools like 360-degree feedback (where team members provide input on your communication style) can help identify areas for improvement.

2. Define Your Leadership Voice

- Do you want to be seen as firm but fair?
- Do you prefer a collaborative and open approach?
- Should your tone be formal or conversational?

Understanding your natural communication tendencies helps you maintain authenticity while adapting to different situations.

3. Establish Core Messages

Determine the key messages you want to consistently convey to your team, such as:

- Your leadership values (e.g., transparency, accountability).
- Your expectations for communication and collaboration.
- Your commitment to team development and success.

SETTING COMMUNICATION GOALS FOR TEAM SUCCESS

Why Communication Goals Matter

Leaders should set clear communication goals to:

- Ensure team members stay informed and engaged.
- Reduce misunderstandings and conflicts.
- Improve collaboration and workflow efficiency.

How to Set Effective Communication Goals

1. Use SMART Goals

SMART (Specific, Measurable, Achievable, Relevant, Time-bound) communication goals create structure and clarity. Examples include:

- Improve team meeting efficiency by keeping discussions under 30 minutes and ensuring all voices are heard.
- Reduce email overload by implementing weekly summaries instead of daily updates.
- Increase feedback loops by conducting quarterly communication check-ins with employees.

2. Define the Purpose of Communication Goals

Ask:

- What challenges does the team face due to poor communication?
- How can better communication enhance productivity and morale?

For instance, if team members feel uninformed about company policies, setting a goal to provide monthly briefings improves clarity.

3. Align Communication Goals with Organizational Objectives

If the organization prioritizes innovation, a communication goal could be:

- Implement open brainstorming sessions where team members share creative ideas without fear of criticism.

If patient-centered care is the focus, a goal might be:

- Train all staff to use empathetic, patient-friendly language in every interaction.

COACHING AND MENTORING FOR COMMUNICATION IMPROVEMENT

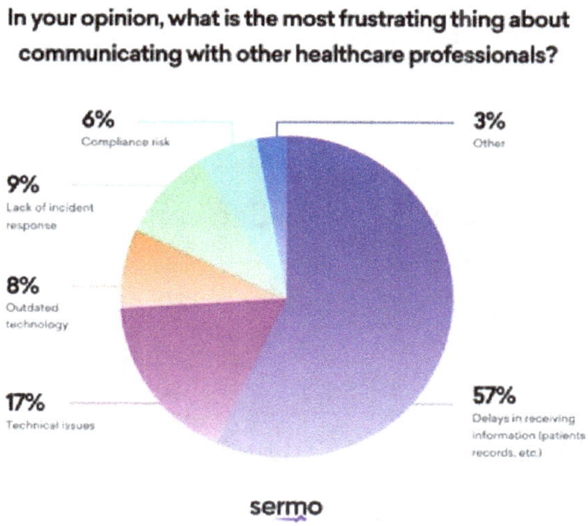

Why Coaching and Mentoring Matter in Leadership Communication

Strong leaders not only improve their own communication skills but also develop their teams through coaching and mentoring.

- Coaching is short-term, focused on skill development and mentoring is long-term, focused on career growth
- Coaching provides constructive feedback on specific task and mentoring offers guidance on overall professional development

- Coaching helps employees improve communication skills quickly and mentoring helps mentees develop a leadership communication style

Strategies for Effective Coaching in Communication

1. Provide Constructive Feedback

Be specific: Instead of "You need to communicate better," say,

"During meetings, try to summarize key points to avoid confusion."

Focus on improvement, not criticism.

2. Encourage Role-Playing

Practicing difficult conversations (e.g., handling conflict, delivering bad news) builds confidence.

3. Offer Training in Active Listening

Leaders should demonstrate and reinforce active listening techniques, such as:

Paraphrasing: "So, what I hear you saying is…"

Asking clarifying questions: "Can you explain what you mean by that?"

EVALUATING TEAM COMMUNICATION EFFECTIVENESS

Why Evaluate Communication?

Without regular evaluation, poor communication habits can go unnoticed, leading to:

- Reduced team cohesion.
- Increased conflicts and misunderstandings.
- Lower productivity and morale.

Methods for Evaluating Communication Effectiveness

1. Team Surveys and Feedback Forms

Ask team members:

- Do you feel heard and valued in meetings?
- Are communication channels effective and accessible?
- Is leadership communication clear and transparent?

2. Monitor Team Interactions

- Observe how well instructions are followed.
- Assess how quickly issues are resolved.

3. Conduct Regular One-on-One Check-ins

- Meet with employees to discuss communication barriers they experience.

CONTINUOUS LEARNING AND ADAPTATION IN LEADERSHIP COMMUNICATION

Why Communication Strategies Must Evolve

Workplaces change constantly, and leaders must adapt their communication styles accordingly.

Strategies for Continuous Learning

1. Stay Updated on Communication Trends
   - Learn about new digital communication tools (e.g., Slack, Microsoft Teams).
   - Attend leadership communication workshops.
2. Embrace Feedback and Self-Reflection
   - Regularly ask for feedback from employees and peers.
   - Reflect on how communication strategies impact team performance.
3. Adjust Communication Methods Based on Team Needs
   - Some teams prefer direct, concise emails, while others benefit from face-to-face meetings.
   - Adapting to different communication preferences fosters better relationships.

MODULE SEVEN

ETHICAL AND LEGAL CONSIDERATIONS IN LEADERSHIP COMMUNICATION

Ethical Leadership v/s Unethical Leadership

Aspects	Ethical Leadership	Unethical Leadership
Decision-making	Prioritize moral values and long-term consequences	Prioritize personal gain or short-term benefits
Transparency	Transparent in their actions and decisions	Hide information or engage in deception
Accountability	Take responsibility for their actions	Blame others or avoid accountability
Employee Well-being	Prioritize the well-being of employees	Exploit or mistreat their workforce
Organisational Culture	Foster a culture of trust and integrity	Create a toxic or unethical work culture

Leadership in healthcare, especially in respiratory care, requires clear, ethical, and legally compliant communication. Leaders must balance transparency with confidentiality, ensuring their communication aligns with ethical principles and legal regulations.

This module explores Understanding ethical communication in healthcare, confidentiality and HIPAA compliance in leadership communication, navigating difficult ethical dilemmas in team management, legal responsibilities of healthcare leaders, and case studies on ethical communication in respiratory care.

UNDERSTANDING ETHICAL COMMUNICATION IN HEALTHCARE

Defining Ethical Communication

Ethical communication in healthcare means:

- Being honest while respecting patient rights.
- Ensuring accuracy in information shared.
- Respecting cultural, religious, and personal values.
- Maintaining patient dignity in all interactions.

Core Principles of Ethical Communication

1. Transparency and Honesty

Leaders must ensure all communication is truthful, clear, and free of misleading information. In respiratory care, this includes:

- Accurately explaining treatment options to patients and families.
- Providing realistic expectations about patient outcomes.

2. Respect for Autonomy

Patients have the right to make informed decisions about their care. Ethical leaders:

- Encourage shared decision-making.
- Ensure patients understand the risks and benefits of procedures.

- Avoid coercive or paternalistic communication.

3. Compassion and Empathy

Patients and their families may be facing stressful and life-changing decisions. Ethical communication requires:

- Active listening to patient concerns.
- Using language that is supportive, not dismissive.
- Providing emotional support while maintaining professional boundaries.

4. Accountability

Leaders must take responsibility for their communication choices and ensure their team follows ethical guidelines. This includes:

- Addressing misinformation immediately.
- Training staff on ethical communication standards.

CONFIDENTIALITY AND HIPAA COMPLIANCE IN LEADERSHIP COMMUNICATION

Why Confidentiality Matters

Healthcare professionals handle sensitive patient information daily. Leaders must ensure that all communication respects patient privacy and complies with the Health Insurance Portability and Accountability Act (HIPAA).

Key HIPAA Compliance Rules

1. The Privacy Rule
   - Protects patients' personal health information (PHI).
   - Requires written patient consent before sharing medical records.
   - Applies to verbal, written, and electronic communications.
2. The Security Rule
   - Requires secure storage and transmission of electronic PHI (ePHI).
   - Leaders must ensure password protection, encryption, and secure access.
3. The Breach Notification Rule
   - Any unauthorized access or disclosure of PHI must be reported.
   - Leaders should have a crisis response plan for data breaches.

Best Practices for Confidential Leadership Communication

1. Secure Internal Communication
   - Use encrypted messaging platforms instead of email for patient discussions.
   - Avoid discussing patient cases in hallways, elevators, or public areas.

2. Educating Staff on Confidentiality
    - Regular HIPAA training ensures all team members understand legal obligations.
    - Conduct role-playing exercises on handling patient information.
3. Proper Handling of Medical Records
    - Ensure only authorized personnel access patient records.
    - Store physical documents in locked cabinets.

Failure to protect patient information can lead to legal consequences, loss of trust, and professional disciplinary actions.

NAVIGATING DIFFICULT ETHICAL DILEMMAS IN TEAM MANAGEMENT

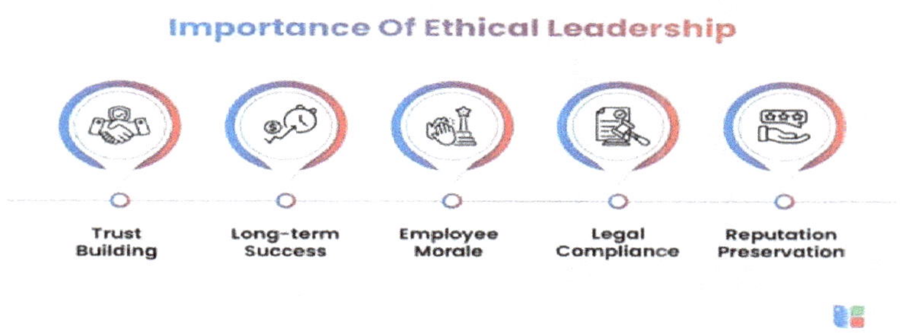
Importance Of Ethical Leadership
Trust Building
Long-term Success
Employee Morale
Legal Compliance
Reputation Preservation

What Are Ethical Dilemmas?

Ethical dilemmas occur when two or more ethical principles conflict, making decision-making complex. In healthcare leadership, these dilemmas often involve:

- Confidentiality vs. patient safety.
- Staff well-being vs. resource allocation.
- Following policies vs. moral obligations.

Common Ethical Dilemmas and Solutions

1. Truth-Telling vs. Avoiding Harm

A patient with a terminal illness asks, "How much time do I have?"

Ethical Response: Provide truthful yet compassionate information. Avoid false hope but maintain emotional support.

2. Staff Conflicts and Ethical Leadership

A respiratory therapist reports a colleague for negligent patient care.

Ethical Response: Investigate the complaint without bias. Uphold professional standards while ensuring fairness.

3. Patient Requests That Challenge Medical Judgment

A patient demands an unnecessary or risky treatment.

Ethical Response: Respect patient autonomy, but provide clear, evidence-based explanations of risks and benefits.

Ethical Decision-Making Framework

To resolve dilemmas, leaders should:

- Identify the ethical conflict.
- Gather all relevant facts.
- Consult policies, legal guidelines, and ethical standards.
- Engage in open discussion with involved parties.
- Make a decision that upholds ethical integrity.

LEGAL RESPONSIBILITIES OF HEALTHCARE LEADERS

Key Legal Duties of Healthcare Leaders

1. Duty of Care

Leaders must ensure safe, high-quality patient care. Negligence or poor communication can lead to malpractice lawsuits.

2. Informed Consent

Before any treatment, patients must:

- Understand all risks, benefits, and alternatives.
- Have the opportunity to ask questions.

3. Workplace Safety Compliance

Leaders must enforce safety regulations to protect staff and patients, including:

- Proper training on infection control.
- Ensuring PPE compliance in respiratory care.

4. Reporting Legal Violations

If leaders witness:

- Medical errors that harm patients.
- Discrimination or harassment in the workplace.
- Violations of HIPAA or safety laws.

They are legally obligated to report these incidents.

Failing to meet legal responsibilities can result in lawsuits, fines, or loss of medical licenses.

CASE STUDIES ON ETHICAL COMMUNICATION IN RESPIRATORY CARE

Case 1: Handling a Data Breach in a Respiratory Care Unit

Situation: A nurse accidentally emails a patient's medical history to the wrong recipient.

Ethical Response:

- Immediately report the breach.
- Inform the patient and relevant authorities.
- Implement stricter email security protocols.

Case 2: Ethical Dilemma in End-of-Life Care

Situation: A terminally ill patient refuses mechanical ventilation, but their family insists.

Ethical Response:

- Respect the patient's autonomy.
- Facilitate a family meeting to discuss medical ethics and patient wishes.
- Offer palliative care alternatives.

Case 3: Addressing Staff Negligence

Situation: A respiratory therapist is found ignoring safety protocols, risking patient health.

Ethical Response:

- Conduct a fair investigation.
- Provide retraining and mentorship.
- If negligence continues, take disciplinary action.

By mastering ethical communication, leaders build trust, integrity, and a strong ethical culture in healthcare.

CONCLUSION

Effective communication is the cornerstone of strong leadership in respiratory care. One of the key takeaways is that communication is not just about conveying information—it is about creating understanding, trust, and alignment. Leaders who actively listen, adapt their communication strategies, and foster open dialogue within their teams create an environment where collaboration thrives. Effective delegation, conflict resolution, and decision-making under pressure all rely on the ability of leaders to communicate with precision and empathy. The book has emphasized the importance of crisis communication and leadership adaptability. Emergencies in respiratory care demand quick thinking, strategic decision-making, and a structured approach to internal and external communication. Effective crisis response not only mitigates immediate risks but also strengthens an organization's resilience for future challenges.

As the healthcare landscape continues to evolve, leaders must commit to continuous learning and adaptation. Exceptional communication skills are what set great respiratory care leaders apart. By integrating the strategies discussed in this book trust-building, crisis management, patient-centered communication, and ethical leadership healthcare professionals can lead with confidence, inspire their teams, and provide the highest level of care to patients. Strong leadership is not just about making decisions it is about communicating those decisions in a way that fosters teamwork, resilience, and positive patient outcomes.

As you continue your journey as a leader in respiratory care, remember that every conversation is an opportunity to lead, inspire, and improve the quality of care. By mastering communication, you will not only enhance your leadership skills but also contribute to a healthier, more connected healthcare environment.

REFERENCES

- American Association for Respiratory Care (AARC). (2020). *Best practices in respiratory care leadership. AARC Publications.*
- Argenti, P. A. (2021). *Strategic communication in business and the professions (8th ed.). McGraw-Hill.*
- Baker, D. P., Day, R., & Salas, E. (2006). *"Teamwork as an essential component of high-reliability organizations."* Health Services Research, 41(4), 1576–1598.
- Bartholomew, K. (2017). *Ending nurse-to-nurse hostility: Why nurses eat their young and each other. Sigma Theta Tau International.*
- Dearing, J. W., & Kreuter, M. W. (2010). *"Designing for diffusion: How can we increase uptake of cancer communication innovations?"* Patient Education and Counseling, 81(S1), S100–S110.
- Edmondson, A. C. (2018). *The fearless organization: Creating psychological safety in the workplace for learning, innovation, and growth*. Wiley.
- Flin, R., O'Connor, P., & Crichton, M. (2008). *Safety at the sharp end: A guide to non-technical skills. CRC Press.*

- Frankel, R. M., & Stein, T. (2013). *Getting to the heart of the matter: Communication and relationships in healthcare. American Academy on Communication in Healthcare.*
- Goleman, D. (2017). Emotional intelligence: *Why it can matter more than IQ. Bantam Books.*
- Marcus, L. J., Dorn, B. C., & McNulty, E. J. (2011). Renegotiating health care: Resolving conflict to build collaboration (2nd ed.). Jossey-Bass.
- Mayfield, J. R., & Mayfield, M. (2017). *"Leader communication strategies: How communication fosters engagement and performance." Journal of Business Communication*, 54(1), 3–24.
- Nembhard, I. M., & Edmondson, A. C. (2006). *"Making it safe: The effects of leader inclusiveness and professional status on psychological safety and improvement efforts in health care teams." Journal of Organizational Behavior*, 27(7), 941–966.
- Nuffield Council on Bioethics. (2009). *Patient safety and ethical concerns in medical communication. Nuffield Council Reports.*
- O'Daniel, M., & Rosenstein, A. H. (2008). *"Professional communication and team collaboration." In R. G. Hughes (Ed.), Patient safety and quality: An evidence-*

based handbook for nurses (pp. 471–494). Agency for Healthcare Research and Quality (AHRQ).

- Patterson, K., Grenny, J., McMillan, R., & Switzler, A. (2012*). Crucial conversations: Tools for talking when stakes are high (2nd ed.)*. McGraw-Hill.
- Reimer, T., & Moore, R. (2021). *Crisis communication in healthcare: Navigating emergencies with clarity and confidence*. Springer.
- Zaccaro, S. J., Rittman, A. L., & Marks, M. A. (2001). *"Team leadership." The Leadership Quarterly,* 12(4), 451–483.

www.ingramcontent.com/pod-product-compliance
Lightning Source LLC
LaVergne TN
LVHW022024200926
848481LV00007B/2530